EATING SMART TO HEALTHY LIFE

Steps to have healthy happy life

Marie Realms

Copyright

Introduction

Eating is not merely a daily ritual; it is a fundamental act that profoundly shapes our lives. The food choices we make impact not only our physical health but also our mental well-being and the quality of our existence. The term "eating smart" signifies a conscientious approach to nourishment, one that empowers us to make choices that are not just satisfying but genuinely life-enhancing.

In this concise Book, we will explore the paramount significance of eating smart. We will unravel the reasons why a thoughtful, informed, and health-conscious approach to our diets is a pivotal key to living a happier, healthier life. As we journey through these pages, we will discover how the foods we consume impact our bodies, our minds, and our overall wellness. By the end, you'll appreciate the profound influence of your dietary choices and, armed with knowledge and insight, you'll be better equipped to make decisions that support a life of vitality and well-being.

Chapter 1: What is nutrition?.

Nutrition is an investigation of what happens in our bodies when we eat certain types of food. This involves examining the composition of the foods including the components; macro and micro nutrients absorbed, used by human beings plus their effects on health. Nutrition, however, lays a solid framework for our general health.

Understanding nutrients

Substances called nutrients are found in food and they feed our bodies. We can categorize these nutrients into two primary groups: macronutrients and micronutrients. These include carbohydrates, fats, and proteins as examples of macronutrients while vitamins and minerals constitute the group of micronutrients.

Nutrition can be considered as one area of health that requires understanding the basic level before making decisions on food we take. This is what enables us to create individualized diet plans, catering to a particular purpose of ours. Besides this, it is vital in matters relating to energy, enlargement, defense against diseases, well being of the mind and others.

The first chapter sets the stage for our
exploration of the realm of nutrition, which
provides the groundwork for our overall physical
condition. This is where informed and healthy
eating choices start coming from in our food
habits

Chapter 2: Building a balanced plate.

The Importance of Portion Control

Portion control is an important aspect that one should consider when looking out for healthy diet. What we feed our bodies, and how much of it we consume, also affects our health. This chapter will outline the importance of portion control and offer some useful tips to prevent you from overeating.

Understanding Portion Control:

1. Adaptation to individual needs

They acknowledge that individuals have distinctive dietary requisites. It accepts that not all people have the same calorie or nutritional needs. One of the most fundamental things in portion control is understanding what your body needs in particular.

2. Avoid Overconsumption:

Eating more than needed can lead to the buildup of unnecessary calories and nutrients not

adequately used by the body. These may result in excessive energy deposition, nutrient imbalance, and associated diseases such as obesity. These risks can be minimized through portion control which promotes moderation.

3. Promote conscious eating:

I linked part control with mindful eating. You get to learn more about whatever you are eating and enjoy it as it comes. By knowing quantities one can tell when they have consumed enough food, avoiding excessive consumption.

4. Managing Weight:

Portion control is therefore a very effective means of controlling or even losing weight for these individuals. Lose weight and maintain good health by eating just enough food.

5. Preventing Nutrient Imbalances:

Eating too much of a certain kind of food can cause essential elements deficiencies. Reducing portion sizes enables you to consume a variety of foodstuff and nutrient rich foods.

6. Enhancing Satisfaction:

Controlling a portion may also increase satisfaction from meals. You should learn how to control your portions and sometimes. a little might be satisfactory because your body has required the exact amount.

It highlights the fact that we differ in body build hence our food portions must also be different. Mindful eating is promoted, controlling weight and avoiding nutrient imbalances. By controlling the portions, we eat according to what our bodies require for optimal health, making us feel better and even aiding in weight management.

Creating a balanced plate .

Balancing nutrients in proportionate quantities is an art which provides needed support for the body. These are some of the key considerations to observe in making balanced and nutrient-rich meals.

1. Start with a board or visual representation:

Just pretend that you have such a plate on your table or, alternatively, imagine a real plate instead of it. You would have an ideal plate if you were to subdivide it into segments representing each food group.

2. Divide a quarter of your plate between lean proteins:

Muscle mass growth, repair, and maintenance require protein. Poultry, fish, lean cuts of meat, tofu, legumes, and beans are considered as lean protein sources. Ensure you choose a suitable protein for your diet needs.

3. Dedicate a quarter of your plate to whole grains:

Carbohydrates for energy are derived from whole grains. Choose alternatives such as brown rice, quinoa, whole wheat pasta and whole wheat bread. Wholegrain has greater fiber content and nutritional value than refined grains.

4. Incorporate Healthy Fats:

Healthy fats might have a direct impact on your health but you will still have to consume them regardless. Include avocados, nuts, seeds and olive oil to your diet. They nourish the brain, aid in absorption of fat soluble vitamins and give long term fuel energy.

5. Don't forget dairy or dairy alternatives:

Incorporate one serving into your meal if you eat dairy and dairy alternatives. Calcium and protein are present in dairy products. Go for low-fat and the fat free ones if you pay attention to your calories.

6. Season with herbs and spices.

Add flavor to your diet by using herbs and spices in your meals that will not add any extra calories or other unhealthy ingredients. Spice up your meals by experimenting with various combinations.

7. Stay Hydrated:

Note also, that drinks are part of your meal, too. Choose water, herbal tea, and other such non calorie drinks. Stick with low sugar drinks and restricted caffeine.

8. Mindful eating:

However, observe mindful eating while consuming your foods. Listen to your body's signals of hunger and satisfaction. It aids in preventing over-consuming while achieving satisfaction with what you eat.

9. Proportions matter:

As you fill your plate, always have in mind proportions.< Although specific sizes will be relative to your own individual case, generally speaking one should aim at making a visually appealing dish consisting of several important ingredients.

Following these guidelines and tailoring them according to your tastes and nutritional demands, you will forever produce balanced diets, which feed your body enough nutrients in correct proportions. Such consideration provides an assurance that the body receives diverse kinds of essential nutrients, keeps one's weight in check as well as manages their energy and general health.

Chapter 3: The Power of Fruits and Vegetable

It's not just about jazzing up the plate by eating multicolored fruits and vegetables. It is a great way to add value to your body. These are also special sets of vitamins, phytochemicals, and dietary nutrients that provide distinct health advantages for every color. Here's how important it is to incorporate these different colors into your diet:

1. Green:

Importance: Chlorophyll is one of the highly potent antioxidants that are found in green vegetables. These also include folate and vitamin K, which are necessary nutrients.

Health benefits:

* Heart health: Research shows that consumption of leafy green vegetables such as spinach, kale and others significantly lowers the risk of heart diseases.

* Bone health: Green vegetables also contain vitamin K that's important for bone health and blood clotting.

* Cancer prevention: Research has shown that there may be compounds in broccoli, kale or any cabbage may help prevent cancers.

2. Red:

Importance: Anthocyanins and lycopene are antioxidants that occur in red fruits and vegetables.

Health benefits:

* Heart health: it showed that eating more tomatoes provided protection against cardiovascular diseases and had a beneficial effect on heart health by reducing the risk of stroke.

* Cancer prevention: Some cancers like prostate cancer can be reduced by some red fruits such as watermelon, and pink grapefruit.

* Skin health: Vitamin C found in red pepper is critical in the formation of collagen and good healthy skin.

3. Orange and Yellow:

Importance: They result from beta-carotene (as a precursor to vitamin A) and other carotenoids.

Health benefits:

* Vision: It boosts amazing sight & eye wellness is beta-carotene.

Immune system: Many orange and yellow fruits have a lot of vitamin C that enhances the body's immune system.

* Skin health: Healthy, glowing skin, which includes carrots and sweet potatoes are these fruits and vegetables.

4. Purple and Blue:

Significance: Inflammation processes are inhibited by anthocyanin from purple and blue colored foods which have strong antioxidant properties.

Health Benefits:

* Brain Health: Anthocyanins are also involved in cognitive function, which has proven useful in preventing Alzheimer's disease.
* Heart Health: Research has proven that an extreme consumption level of blueberries is able to lower the risk of Cardiovascular disease.
* Anti-Aging: Antioxidants present in these foods help to reduce oxidative stress that leads to the speedy process of ageing.

5. White:

Significance: Allicin and other phytonutrients can be found in vegetables like cauliflower and garlic.

Health Benefits:

* Heart Health: Allicin may reduce the chances of having a heart attack in a coronary artery.
* Cancer Prevention: Some few varieties of such white vegetables would even protect people from certain types of cancer.
Bone Health: Cauliflower and garlic are a great source of potassium and magnesium.

The Significance of Variety:

* Balanced Nutrition: This shows that eating different coloured foods will give you diverse types of vitamins, minerals and antioxidants which will make your diet balanced.

* Reduced Risk of Chronic Diseases: Consuming a color diet can reduce the risk of developing such illnesses as obesity, cardiac disorders, cancer, and diabetes among others.

* Enhanced Immunity: Eating fruits and vegetables keeps you safe from infections.

* Anti-Inflammatory Properties: They could contain a distinct anti-inflammatory compound, which helped fight against inflammation. Eating multicolored is not only about making food look good but also it means getting the numerous and complimentary body health advantages that each of these colors come with. You should try and put a rainbow on your plate just like in nature because this is what nature gives you and not the other way round.

Chapter 4: Protein Source

Why choose lean protein sources?

- **Several reasons make it necessary to select lean protein sources. Firstly, it promotes healthy living since it provides the basic components that help in effective functioning of the body and hence the healthy condition. Here's why opting for lean protein sources is important:**

- **Weight Management: Most lean protein sources are low on calories. They make you stay full for a long period of time thus cutting down total calories consumed.**

- **Heart Health: Consumption of saturated fat should be reduced as it affects heart health. Skinless poultry, lean cuts of meats, and plant sources provide more lean proteins with lesser saturated fats than those high in fats.**

- **Muscle Maintenance: Muscles need protein for their repair or repair after injury and during growth. Lean protein options provide you with the needed amount of protein without excess fat taken up. This is especially critical for people involved in physical training, exercise or hard work.**

- **Blood Sugar Control:** Some lean proteins can be consumed in moderation and this may assist in stabilizing blood sugar. These products possess a low GI and are less likely to result into sudden fluctuation of blood glucose levels hence recommended for people with diabetes and those in danger of developing it.

- **Digestive Health:** Fatty proteins are difficult for the body to process and they cause stomach discomfort. It is gentler on one's digestive system.

Plant-Based Proteins:

It also comes with popularity, being healthier and environmentally friendly than other sources of protein. Here's why they are significant:

Nutrient Density: Plant-based protein sources contain a wealth of healthy substances such as fiber, vitamins, and minerals. For example, legumes are loaded with protein and other vital minerals.

Lower Saturated Fat: Plant-based sources of protein normally contain no saturated fats and are also free of cholesterol. These supplements may be beneficial in reducing the risk of heart disease and maintaining good cardiovascular function.

Reduced Environmental Impact: Plant products are usually more environmentally friendly than other animal-sourced ones. Selecting plant based protein contributes to sustainability and reducing number of greenhouse gases.

Diverse Protein Sources: There are multiple proteins in plant-based eating such as dry beans, lentils, tofu, tempeh, nuts, seeds, and whole grain cereals available. The variation offers you chance to have different tastes and multiple nutrients.

Flexibility: plant-based proteins are flexible and can fit in different meals depending on the dietary needs such as the vegetarian, vegan, or filter diets.

Inflammation reduction: diets rich in plant-based protein, especially high antioxidant foods may assist to decrease body inflammation contributing towards overall good health.

On the other hand, it is important to ensure that there is variety when choosing plant proteins and take in all essential amino acid and minerals by the body system. Different types of plants may be used as protein sources for an individual to achieve wholesome protein enriched diet. However, a balanced meal should incorporate only the right kind of lean protein sources available from animals as well as plants. These proteins are usually known as the thin ones which are connected to losing some weight, taking care of heart system, assisting the muscles, and regulating a normal sugar balance. However, plant proteins are also nutrient dense, sustainable, and multiple protein sources, making them essential for any dietary plan.

Chapter 5: Carbohydrates

****Understanding the Role of Carbohydrates in Energy Production:**

- The other important type of dietary components is carbohydrates which are among the crucial macronutrients. The body's main, as well as the most reliable source of energy is then the understanding of role of carbohydrates concerning the maintenance of a balanced and healthy diet.

- Energy Source: The body, breaks down carbohydrates, into glucose (sugar). For example, it utilizes glucose as the preferred source of energy for multiple bodily functions like physical activities, as well as cognitive processes.

- Glycogen Storage: The liver and muscles store excess glucose as glycogen. The reserves act as reservoirs of instant energy which can be utilized when the body becomes more active.

- Brain Fuel: The brain uses glucose as its main source of energy. Carbohydrate intake must be maintained on a regular basis in order for the brain to function at its best level so as to keep the mind clear, focused, and have optimal cognitive skills.

- Workout Fuel: Carbohydrates are essential for muscle glycogen repletion in sports persons as well as active people and help power work out routines as well as enhance exercise performances. Therefore, these glycogen storage are key in endurance activities.

- Blood Sugar Regulation: Eating carbohydrate rich fiber foods like bran products, pulses, fruits and leafy green vegetables aid in regulating blood glucose concentrations. Due to this fact, fiber delays glucose uptake that prevents glucose peaks and troughs.

Choosing Healthy Carbs:

- Whole Grains: Eat foods made of whole grains such as brown rice, quinoa, whole-wheat bread, and oats. These whole grains are unrefined which means that they have more fiber, vitamins, and minerals compared to other refined grains.

- Fruits: Fruits are nature's forms of carbs, which contain vitamins, minerals, fibers, and antioxidants. Take different types of fruit in order to obtain all possible minerals and micronutrients.

- Vegetables: Such examples include leafy greens like spinach and kale which have few carbs but many nutrients and fiber along with the other vegetables like broccoli and pepper. It has been effective in controlling high levels of blood sugar, as well as the feeling of satiation.

- Legumes: An example is that the diet contains more fibre and protein in the case of beans, lentils and peas. They provide a steady flow of power and aid in digestion as well.

- Nuts and Seeds: It houses several valuable reservoirs of fatty oil, protein, and carbohydrate. They can work as good snacks and provide lasting energy.

- Minimize Refined Carbs: Control intakes of food and beverages with added sugars, refined grains, or large processed carbohydrates. This can cause fluctuation in energy, weight gain and potential problems with other health conditions.

- Complex Carbohydrates: Go for simple carbohydrates, which are short-chained sugars. Their absorption into their body is gradual, and the energy flows slowly. Items such as wheat, beans,

**potatoes, and other similar foods form
part of these.**

●   **This is where you select healthful
carbohydrates that offer nutrition with
high-fiber which supports energy
production, stabilizes the blood sugar
level as well as general fitness. Include
various types of carbohydrates in your
diet in this manner so that you can
benefit from each and every nutrient
they contain.**

Chapter 6:Fats: Good Fats vs. Bad Fats

**Different Types of Dietary Fat: **

Fat is an important part of our nutrition offering energy as well as other functions within our bodies. listade2. Nevertheless, fats are not identical. There are three main types of dietary fat, each with its own distinct characteristics and effects on health:

1. Saturated Fats:

*Source: Mostly we found saturated fats in animal products including beef and pork, butter, cheese and many others types of dairies. Some of these metals are found in some tropical oils such as coconut oil and palm oil.

- *Properties: Their chemical structure is without any double bond leading to a situation where we can call them "saturated fats".

*Health Risks: The high intake of saturated fats results to heart diseases being susceptible. These are able to increase LDL (bad) cholesterol in the blood and result in plague forming.

2. Unsaturated Fats:

- *Types: However, unsatisfied fats fall in two broad groupings, which are mono-unsaturated and poly-unsaturated fats.

- *Sources: Olive oil, avocados and nuts contain mono-unsaturated fats. Omega-3 and omega-6 fatty acids such as those in fatty fish, flaxseed, soybean oil and corn oil are examples of polyunsaturated fats.

- *Properties: unsaturated fats have one or more double bond that makes an irregular angle in the fatty acid chain.

*Health Benefits: These are called unsaturated fats that lower blood cholesterol and which, therefore, are called good. Omega-3 specifically is one of those fats with anti-inflammatory actions important for brain and retina wellness.

3. Trans Fats:

- *Source: The main source of trans-fat is hydrogenated oil, an artificial fat that makes oils solid at lower temperatures. They were often found in partially hydrogenated vegetable oils as well as many processed, deep-fried goods.

- *Properties: Trans fats are structurally analogous to saturated fats and are hard at room temperatures.

*Health Risks: In terms of adverse impact on health, trans fats are probably the worst type of fat. It also leads to an elevation in LDL and decrease in HDL which makes them susceptible to coronary heart disease. In addition, they are linked to inflammations and other health problems.

**The Differences and Health Risks: **

Saturated fat is often hard at room temperature and predominantly comes from animals' products such as meat, milk, cheese, eggs and lard. Excess consumption is associated with cardiovascular diseases.

Unsaturated fats are usually liquid at ordinary temperatures and may help protect the heart by replacing the saturated fats in nutrition. These supply the body with essential fats, which possess numerous advantages on health.

The most damaging is a trans fat,which mainly can be found in ready-made food products. The former can cause higher levels of bad cholesterols leading to heart problems. Some nations even implemented policies aimed at banning or reducing the levels of trans fats in the food supply.

It is necessary to control saturated and trans fat intake and, instead, increase the consumption of unsaturated fats for a healthy living. Using unsaturated fats like olive oil and fat fish instead of saturated ones improves cardiac health and general state of organism.

.

Source of healthy fats:
Sources of Healthy Fats and Their Benefits:

Fat is an essential part of any healthy diet and has numerous benefits for your whole body. Here are some sources of healthy fats and the advantages they provide:

1. Avocado:

- - *Healthy Fat Type: * Monounsaturated fat.

Benefits:
- - Heart Health: These include reducing the levels of bad cholesterols hence preventing the chances of heart attacks.

- - Nutrient Density: Fiber, folate, fiber, vitamin K, mineral, antioxidant — avocado has a lot of these.

- - Skin and Eye Health: Areas are high in lutein and zeaxanthin (good for skin and eyes).

**2. Fatty Fish (Salmon, Mackerel, Sardines): **

- - *Healthy Fat Type: * Omega-3 polyunsaturated fat.

- *Benefits:*
- - Heart Health: They include omega-3 fatty acids that lower triglyceride levels

and curb the production of
inflammatory products.

- - Brain Health: Omega-3 is important
for preventing age related cognitive
decline and maintaining normal brain
function.

- - Joint Health: They can also reduce
symptoms that accompany
inflammations like for example
arthritis.

**3. Nuts (Almonds, Walnuts, Pecans): **

- - *Healthy Fat Type: Monounsaturated
and polyunsaturated fats.

- *Benefits:*
- - Heart Health: It appears that eating
nuts reduces the risk of heart disease.

- - Weight Management: Nuts are also
very dense in calories, but they can
make one feel fuller leading to more
controlled weights.

- - Antioxidants: Generally, whole nuts
contain antioxidants and other
beneficial substances promoting one's
overall health.

4. Olive Oil:

- *Healthy Fat Type: * Primarily monounsaturated fat

- *Benefits:

- Heart Health: Olive oil serves as one of the primary components in the Mediterranean diet, which is linked to reduced cases of heart ailments.

- Anti-inflammatory: Prevention of inflammation and chronic diseases risk.

- Skin Health: Olive has a good form of oleic acid that benefits the skin and could prevent UV radiation.

5. Flaxseeds:

- *Healthy Fat Type: Omega-3 polyunsaturated fat (ALA).

- *Benefits:*

- Heart Health: Flaxseed may also help lower blood pressure and decrease risks of cardiovascular diseases.

- Digestive Health: These can serve as dietary fiber that may assist in the functioning of the digestive system.

- Omega-3 Fatty Acids: Taking fruits and vegetables only serves as a good diet plan, and you should add extra omega-3s which are obtainable from flax seeds.

**6. Dark Chocolate (in moderation): **

- - *Healthy Fat Type: Saturation monounsaturated.

- *Benefits:*
- - Heart Health: Studies show that there is a link between dark chocolate and lowering of blood pressure as well as good effect on the heart system.lea

- - Antioxidants: Flavonoids which have good health benefits that are potent antioxidants.

- - Mood Enhancement: Dark chocolates containing mood boosters.

7. Coconut:

- *Healthy Fat Type: These are the saturated fats, mainly as lauric acid.

- *Benefits:*

- Weight Management: The coconut might help in weight loss, as MCTs can increase calorie burning as it enhances energy expenditure.

- Brain Health: These are suggested to hold the best brain health effects and

hence considered as super-fats by some
people.

- **Skin and Hair Health: Many cultures use coconut oil for its skin and hair benefits.**

The use of multiple sources for such healthy fats could give you many health benefits. These fats are good but remember they contain a lot of calories. The concept of balance lays the foundation for a balanced diet.

Chapter 7: Hydration and the role of water

The Significance of Staying Well-Hydrated for Overall Health:

It is important to stay hydrated because staying healthy involves proper nutrition which requires one to be well hydrated. The importance of water cannot be stressed too far as it is virtually involved in most body functions.

1.**Cell Function: Cell functions are highly dependent on water which delivers nutrients and oxygen while collecting waste.

2.**Digestive Health: Enough water helps to facilitate the digestive process by breaking down the food and moving it through the digestive system. It prevents issues like constipation

3.**Temperature Regulation: This water plays a crucial role in adjusting body temperatures. This aids in cooling and dissipation of heat produced by the body, particularly during physical exercise and in an atmosphere.

4.**Cognitive Function: Cognitive function may be impeded as a result of dehydration through effects on concentration, alertness, and short-term memory.

5. **Joint Lubrication: Joint hydration ensures they are well-lubricated hence reduces the likelihood of developing joint pain or injury.

6.**Detoxification: Water flushes out toxins by way of urine and sweat.

7.**Skin Health: Hydrated skin is smooth, soft and without any scaling on it. However, dry or scaly skin may lead to prematurely aged skin. To enhance hydrated skin with a youthful look and fresh appearance, water needs to be taken properly.

8.**Heart Health: ** Dehydration puts a stress on the cardiovascular system causing a high pulse and low blood volume.

**Guidelines for Daily Water Intake: **

Daily water take depends on the age, gender, lifestyle, and climatic environments. Commonly referred to as "eight times of eight glasses", the "8x8" rule emphasizes that one should drink eight 8-ounce glasses every day, making about two liters. Here are some general recommendations.

1.**The National Academies of Sciences, Engineering, and Medicine: Men could take this quantity which is almost up to 4 liters on a daily basis while the woman takes this quantity which is almost up to 4 liters on a daily basis.

2. **Individual Needs: For instance, physical activity, climate, and individual health conditions will influence your water needs. You will require more water to balance the loss of fluids as a result of sweating in warm weather and upon engaging in vigorous activities.

3. **Thirst as a Guide: Trust your body's natural thirst as an indicator of when you need water. Drink if you are thirsty and listen to your body. The best way that indicates you are drinking enough water in case your urine is pale yellow.

4. **Hydrating Foods: However, remember that most are composed of water, for instance, fruits and vegetables will also count to your daily water intake. Eating foods having high-water content like watermelon, cucumber, and orange complements drinking fluids.

5. **Individual Variations: The most crucial thing is how well you know yourself and what you need. Adjust your water intake depending on what your body says. Others will need more water.

Always bear in mind that people have different water needs and these vary on a daily basis also.

Maintain an equilibrium of input and output fluids but sufficient hydration should be done based on one's state of health..

Recognizing the signs of dehydration is essential to take prompt action and rehydrate to maintain your health. Here are common signs and symptoms of dehydration:

1.**Thirst: When your body is thirsty, it's simply giving the signal that you need more water. It is normally one of the first indicators that a person has become dehydrated.

2.**Dark Urine: Dehydration is indicated by concentrated urine which can appear either dark yellow or as amber-colored urine. Healthy and properly hydrated urine should appear pale yellow.

3.**Reduced Urination: If you're going fewer times and passing little amounts, this could mean that you're developing a state of dehydration.

4.**Dry Mouth and Dry Skin: The mouth could have a dry or sticky sensation while the skin may seem to be very tight. They may also get their lips chapped or even lose skin's clasticity.

5.**Fatigue and Weakness: Dehydration may result in hypotension due to insufficient perfusion of necessary organs resulting in tiredness and weakness.

6.**Dizziness and Lightheadedness: When fluid volume is poor, there could be diminished blood pressure, and the person may experience dizziness or faintness when standing after sitting.

7.**Headache: Headaches may occur due to reduced blood flow leading to dehydration and less oxygen in the brain itself.

8.**Rapid Heartbeat: The body then increases the heart rate leading to dehydration which decreases the blood volume.

9.**Dry or sticky mucus membranes: This results in dry mucus membrane in the nose and throat, which might be unpleasant and makes one vulnerable to various infections.

10.**Muscle Cramps: Dehydration affects the equilibrium of electrolytes within the body therefore causing cramps especially during a workout.

11. **Sunken Eyes: In serious situations of dehydration, eyes can appear as being sunken in and skin turgor may be lost.

12. **Mental Changes: Cognitive function could be affected by dehydration that may cause problems with concentration, irritability, or some degree of confusion.

13. **Fainting: People become unconscious, experience dizziness after severe dehydration when their blood pressure falls down.

Immediately, one needs to treat dehydration through drinking of fluids. Water is better; however, some oral rehydration solutions or beverages with electrolytes are good alternatives when it comes to vigorous physical work or excess fluid drainage. For severe dehydration or persistent symptoms, seek immediate medical care. Severe dehydration can be treated using different interventions.

Chapter 8: Practical Tips for Healthy Eating

Mindful Eating: Strategies for Being More Aware of What and How You Eat

Mindful eating is an exercise where one should pay maximum attention to the process of consumption, which includes tasting and feeling the food on the tongue. It could be useful for building a better rapport with meals, avoiding overeating, and experiencing the deliciousness of them in a wholesome manner. Here are strategies for being more mindful when you eat:

Eat Without Distractions: Switch off the television set, turn around your phone and do not work or read while eating. Pay attention only to what you are eating, thus better enjoying the flavor and signs of your body.

Engage Your Senses: Do not forget to observe the looks of your meal before taking it, pay attention to its taste and feel it with your tongue. Take note of the colors, forms, and aroma. It improves the sensory pleasure of food.

Chew Slowly: You help yourself to swallow food by chewing slowly for as long as possible and thus facilitating proper digestion. It helps your body tell that it's full so that you don't overeat.

**Mindful Portion Control: Always avoid large portions. Serve smaller portions initially, use smaller plates in order to help control portion sizes. If you are not yet full, there is always a chance to have some more.

**Sip Water: In order to help you eat slowly, take a sip of water after every bite.

**Check-in with Hunger and Fullness:

Take a break in between your meals to check how full you feel. Eat till you feel no longer hungry but not stuffed.

**Practice Gratitude: Before you eat, remember to honor and give thanks for the food that will be enjoyed. This could cultivate a healthy outlook towards food and nurture healthy eating habits.

Avoid Emotional Eating: Take control over how your mind is feeling during food consumption. Do not seek food as a way of comforting your emotional crags or loneliness; rather try alternative methods of dealing with such sentiments.

**Plan Nutritious Meals in Advance: **

**Meal Prep: For instance, one can prepare a meal plan for a week by creating the ingredient list, planning ahead of time, and storing some healthy ready-made food in order not to go for less healthy alternatives when it is close.

**Balanced Meals: Include lean proteins, whole grains, lots of vegetables, and healthier fats. Therefore, you will be assured of various nutrients and a delectable blend of flavors.

**Snacks: However, try and prepare healthy snacks such as cut vegetables, fresh fruit, and maybe a handful of nuts to help your hunger pangs in between meals.

**Stay Hydrated: Ensure that you have water available. When taking conscious eating seriously, one must ensure proper hydration because sometimes a person who feels dehydrated might think they feel hungry rather than thirsty.

**Mindful Grocery Shopping: Make a checklist of what foodstuffs you decide to have at home when going out shopping for groceries. Make sure you follow this checklist when experiencing food cravings and avoid any unhealthier types of food.

By following this strategy and adopting it in your eating habits, you'll be able to avoid junk foods as well as mindfully eat healthy. It may thus lead to effective digestion, reduce overeating and generally put one in good spirits.

**Guidance on Making Healthy Choices When Dining at Restaurants and Eating Out Smart: **

Visiting restaurants is indeed enjoyable but always poses difficulties in the selection of healthy meals. Here are some tips to help you dine out wisely while still enjoying your meal:

1. Plan Ahead:

- **Review the Menu in Advance: Several eateries publish their menus on their websites. Check the menu prior to going to the restaurant for healthier alternatives instead of giving-in to unhealthy options on sight.

2. Watch Portion Sizes:

- **Share or Take Half Home: Some restaurant portions are actually far bigger than what you require in a single meal. It is better to share your meal with another person or request take away from the beginning, leaving half of the food for later.

**3. Choose Healthier Cooking Methods: **

- **Opt for Grilled or Steamed: Opt for dishes which are roasted, steamed or baked instead of those that are fried or deep-fried. Therefore, there will be fewer fats added to your food.

4. Customize Your Order:

- **Ask for Modifications: Feel free to add dressing of your choice, order a sandwich with whole grains, or request extra side veggies. A majority of the restaurants are trying to meet customers' unique needs.

**5. Be Mindful of Sauces and Dressings:

- **Ask for sauces on the Side: Several of these sauces and dressings are extremely caloric and fatty. Tell them off the side as you manage your intake.

6. Control Your Appetizers:

- **Choose Wisely: Prefer healthy starters such as salad or vegetables rather than deep-fried or cheese. It will enable you to kickstart your meal correctly.

**7. Be Mindful of Beverages: **

- **Drink Water: Go for water or herbal tea or other low calorie drinks as alternatives to sugar filled sodas or high calorie cocktails

8. Limit Bread and Chips:

**Don't Fill Up on Bread: Although tempting to eat the free bread/chips, do not exceed yourself and leave some space for your main course meal.

9. Practice Portion Control:

**Split the Dish: When you decide to have a large entree, you should either share the meal with another person or package the other portion and eat it at home as soon as possible.

**10. Pay Attention to Your Body: **

Eat slowly. Enjoy every bite you take, chewing carefully. That will help your body to see that it is already full and hence protect your body from oversupply.

11. Choose Desserts Wisely:

**Share or Opt for Fruit: Just desserts! – If you have dessert, share it with others on your table. Otherwise, find fruit options or smaller servings.

12. Mind Your Portions:

Avoid Super-Sizing: Such meals are usually super-sized, and this is what causes excessive eating in restaurants. Stick to regular portions.

13. Listen to Your Body:

**Stop When Satisfied: Listen carefully to both hunger and satiety signals of your body. Stop eating when you're full, no matter how much food is still there on your plate.

14. Avoid All-You-Can-Eat Options:

**Limit Buffets: Over-eating could be encouraged by all you can eat buffets. Opt for

fruits and vegetable salads if you have to eat in a
buffet joint.

15. Practice Moderation:

**Indulge Occasionally: It is fine to have some
less healthy ones occasionally but make sure they
are consumed in portions and combined with
other wholesome foods for the rest of the time.

These strategies are useful in helping you order
wisely from restaurants menu while ensuring
that you still practice healthy living.

Chapter 9: Special Diets and Considerations

Navigating Special Dietary Needs, Restrictions, and Allergies:

Therefore, it is important for you to choose carefully what foods you will eat, while communicating well with those around you. Whether you have dietary restrictions due to health concerns, allergies, or personal choices, here are some tips to help you manage your specific dietary needs:

1. Educate Yourself:

Ensure you understand yourself well enough on what you need in terms of food or whatever it is that does not work for you. Get information on what types of foods (especially which ingredients, foods, and food groups) are good or bad for your health.

**2. Read labels and menus:

Ensure to read food labels carefully while shopping for groceries to determine the presence of allergens and/or ingredients which should be avoided. When eating at a restaurant, request the list of ingredients or an allergy menu.

3. Communicate Clearly:

Inform a restaurant manager regarding your food preferences and if you have any problems like allergies. Provide details about your needs and inquire regarding food-preparation procedures.

4. Carry Snacks:

Carry with you safe and convenient snacks, particularly in case of possible allergic reactions while traveling. This allows you an alternative source of safe food when it may not readily be available.

**5. Plan Meals in Advance: **

As much as possible, prepare your meals and snacks ahead of time. The probability is then reduced that one goes out of business with no alternatives.

6. Cook at Home:

In this way, cooking your own meal gives you full confidence that the allergens will never get through accidentally and that no "cheat" food is used.

7. Inform friends and family:

Tell them about any special requirements on your menus such as avoiding certain foods due to allergies or personal preferences. They do this to prepare adequately while hosting parties or cooking for you.

.

8. Explore Substitutes:

Analyze and practice on an alternative option to some of the avoided ingredients. Such as the dairy-free or gluten-free substitutes.

**9. Carry an allergy card.

When embarking on overseas travels, carry one allergy card per language spoken locally. It also enables you to let people you will be communicating with in other countries about your dietary limitations.

10. Seek Support:

- Participate in diet support groups, or online communities of those with similar dietary restrictions and/or allergies. They sometimes give meaningful advice and moral support.

**11. Be Cautious When Dining Out: **

- Select restaurants that arc known for being customer friendly and catering for people who require special diets. Make sure the cheese for your meal gets made under safe conditions. Talk to the chef or manager about this.

12. Emergency Preparedness:

- In case you suffer severe hypersensitivity reaction always carry your hypersensitivity medications e.g., epi-pen or antihistamines). Make sure everyone who will be using a fire extinguisher knows how to do so in an emergency situation.

13. Stay Informed:

- Monitor changes, the development of updated food labeling regulations as well as introduction of foods suitable to your dieting plans.

14. Be Patient:

- Remember, managing dietary restrictions or allergies can be difficult. Patiently adjust to your own circumstances, and others'.

**15. Consult a Healthcare Professional: **

- Always seek consultation of a registered dietitian or a healthcare professional specialized and knowledgeable about your food sensitivity issues or for specific health problems.

While following a special dietary regime, having some restrictions, or suffering from one or more allergic reactions may not be easy, with thorough precautions and proper information exchange, you still may feel well and eat healthily at the same time.

Guidance for Those Following Plant-Based Eating Plans (Vegetarian and Vegan Diets):

A plan is also required whereby one has to take in some form of a vegetable or even vegan diet as it could be good for the body and heart but not some few things. Here's guidance for those on plant-based eating plans:

**1. Diversify Your Food Choices: **

Consume a variety of fruits and vegetables to get several vitamins/nutritional and mineral values. Other foods that belong in this category are fruits, vegetables, legumes, whole grains, nuts, beans, soy based-food such as tofu and tempeh.

**2. Ensure Sufficient Protein Intake: **

This is key since it boosts proteins which ensure that one as a whole remains healthy and his/ her muscles. To increase on nutrients and decrease on carbohydrates, you can consider taking pulses like chickpeas, beans, lentils, peanuts, or quinoa.

**3. Pay Attention to Iron: **

For example, this consists of iron obtained from foods such as lentils, tofu, chickpeas, and breakfast cereals. Put them all in one bowl made of strawberries, green peppers and oranges, mix then combine with other iron-containing foods such as fish, spinach, beans and liver.

4. Focus on Calcium:

Calcium is implicated in general bone problems, cancer, and even cardiovascular issues. Set plant milk substitutes with an extra nutrient like kale, collaborate leaf greens, and Ca-set tofu.

**5. Get Adequate Vitamin B12: **

In another word, there is a shocking fact that animal-related foods have the main reservoir of vitamin B12. On the other hand, vegans can only consume vitamin B12 through taking supplements or eating special foods like soy milk, cereals, grain or a few yeast extracts.

6. Include healthy fats:

These are foods containing good oils like avocados, nuts, and seeds; or simply other health oils. Therefore, it has pushed that healthy unsaturated fats be encouraged.

7. Omega-3 Fatty Acids:

Flax seeds, chia seeds, walnuts, and hemp seeds contain plant based omega-3s. These healthy fats are also essential for cardiovascular and cranial health.

8. Whole grains are key.

Eat more whole grains such as brown rice, quinoa, whole wheat and oats and not refined carbohydrates to maintain a healthy diet.

9. Don't Overlook Fiber:

Digestion and health through fiber in plant-based diets. Consume an adequate amount of fibrous food including fruits, vegetables, whole grain wheat or legumes.

**10. Carefully Choose Fortified Foods: **

There are some nutrients such as vitamin D, calcium and B12 that one can obtain from fortified plant based drink and cereal breakfast.

**11. Explore Plant-Based Protein Sources: **

Add flavor to your cuisine by incorporating seitan, tempeh, edamame or different kinds of beans which are made of plant protein.

12. Meal Planning:

Ensure that you prepare your meals ahead of time in order to see daily improvement on nutritional grounds. In this way, it helps to keep at bay the habit of feeding randomly, thereby ensuring that there will be something good available to eat at all times.4

13. Learn to Cook:

Plant based diet dictates for individuals to be in a position to boil vegetables and fruits. The recipes are varied, you can make delicious and healthy meals according to your taste and preferences.

14. Stay Hydrated:

Drink lots of water to remain healthy.

15. Be Informed:

This includes new information about plant-based, healthy foods, and their suggestions. Another good reference can be found on book websites and other sites including certified registered dietitians, who specialize on plant's based diets.

.

16. Listen to Your Body:

On the other hand, it is essential to note that it could result in stomach upsets sometimes when one consumes such foods. If you experience any weird feelings, consult a doctor.

Some plant diets may indeed fall short of the nutrients required by the body, including micronutrients and macronutrients. For example, you can search for 'vegetable-based nutrition specialized' in one of the registered dieticians online and have a personalized consultation about your health conditions through losing weight or eating healthy.

**Considerations for Individuals on Gluten-Free
and Low-Carb Diets: **

There are also individuals who follow gluten-
free/low carb diets with specific food
requirements. Here are some key considerations
for each:

Gluten-Free Diet:

**Celiac Disease and Non-Celiac Gluten
Sensitivity: Persons with celiac disease and
NCGS are not allowed even to consume wheat,
barley, rye and their products.

**Gluten-Free Labeling: In case of doubts the
label "gluten free" should be looked for this
standard concerns on the maximum content of
the gluten. Lastly, it will prevent cross-
contamination and/or unintentional exposure
during gluten.

**Cross-Contamination: Ensure that there are
no cross contaminations at home and the
restaurant kitchens. Use different cooking
devices and surfaces to avoid cross
contamination.

**Fiber Intake: This situation arises because
some of the foods rich in fiber such as wheat
contain gluten. Also have some of them, fruits,
veggies, legumes and the gluten free whole grains
like quinoa, brown rice etc.

**Nutrient Balance: Always check in nutrient balance. Gluten-free diets do not provide all essential nutrients like B vitamins, iron and fiber. You should try the fortified gluten free as well as a gluten free multivitamin if necessary.

Low-Carb Diet:

**Carbohydrate Sources: Low-carb diet is a specific diet in which an individual has to cut down carbohydrates intake to lose weight or in case of diabetic management. Eat non starchy vegetables, nuts, seeds, fruits, and a low fat diary. Also eat unprocessed meat like chicken and fish.

**Dietary Fiber: On the other hand, if you want your body to digest properly and hence feel great, ensure that even if you embrace a low-carb diet, you consume foods that are rich in fiber. As an example, avocados, flaxseeds, and leafy greens are good choices.

**Healthy Fats: Consume more of the healthy fats including avocados, olive oil, nuts, and fatty fish. Some people even considered teaching Fridays because they could use healthy fats that would give suitable energy level and satiety for low carb diet. page: 30 words: 296

**Protein Intake: Consider adding a lean protein since it is good at maintaining muscle while undergoing a weight loss process.[...]

**Electrolytes: Increase your dietary intake of potassium to ward off excess losses of electrolytes as you cut carbs down.

**Monitor blood sugar: Ensure you take more care of yourself especially in case you diabetes or undertake a low carb diet. In certain instances low carb may not prove appropriate for blood-glucose regulation purposes.

.

**Long-Term Sustainability: Consider whether you will feel good about following such a low-carb diet next year or in five years' time. Select a diet plan which provides important vitamins for losing weight.

**Seek professional advice: For example, in special health cases or extreme diet modifications, it is recommendable for one to obtain medical advice as well consulting a dietician to include the right amount of necessary vitamins.

Ensure you do not take up sugar, but eat nutritive unprocessed food during either gluten free or low carb dieting. In some cases these diets have been known to work well with some health issues, however taking a healthcare provider or a registered dietitian would make this safer for oneself.

Chapter 10: Staying on Track and Setting Goals

Tools and Strategies for Monitoring Your Diet and Health Journey:

Keeping track of your diet and health journey is essential as it helps you make informed choices towards realizing set goals. Here are some tools and strategies to help you track your progress effectively:

**1. Food Journal or App: **

Maintain a food diary in which you document all of your intakes including foods, drinks, etc. You can also track your food using a nutrition tracking app like MyFitnessPal or Cronometer. These tools can tell you how much calories you take in every day, the balance of macros, and also the micro nutrients that you consume.

2. Portion Control:

Use of measuring cups, a food scale or portion control plates for accurate management of serving sizes. This way, you will not eat a lot which is a good thing because when one eats too much it can cause health problems.

3. Body Measurements:

Ensure that you are regularly taking and tracking your body weight, body fat percentage, waist circumference, etc. It gives another perspective about what you have done apart from just using the scale.

4. Photos:

Take the pictures of your before and after body change for visual documentation of the transformation. It can be motivational seeing your progress through comparing photos.

5. Blood Tests:

Ensure that you visit a healthcare provider for blood tests depending on your health objectives aimed at indicating cholesterol levels, glucose, and nutrient status. Such simple routine examinations could reveal trends of your health.

6. Physical Activity Tracker:

You may also use a fitness tracker, a smart phone application or any other system to measure your level of activity. They enable you to create activity targets, count the number of steps walked, distance, and calories burnt, and also monitor your heart rate.

7. Habit-Tracking Apps:

Track your habits using apps such as HabitBull and Habitica for making positive changes in your life. Here, you will be able to make set goals such as those involving the intake of healthy foods, exercises, and various other health behaviors.

8. Self-Reflection and Journaling:

Make sure you record your progress, struggles and victories in a journal. You can use this to detect diet-related patterns and emotions in your health and wellness journeys.

9. Calorie Counting:

To maintain your caloric focus, use a daily calorie-counter app to record what and how much you eat and to track your progress towards your daily calorie goals.

10. Goal Setting:

Come up with SMART goals like setting a timeframe for the diet plan, selecting relevant diets and a diet regime you can achieve. Ensure to regularly evaluate and make changes where necessary, on these goals.

11. Support Groups:

- Become a member of an online or local group on healthy eating or lifestyle objectives. You may find this motivation or education when you share your experiences and achievements with others.

**12. Wellness Coach or Registered Dietitian: **

Work with a wellness coach or a dietician that
will give you feedback on how you are doing and
advice according to what you need.

13. Mindfulness and Meditation:

Practice mindfulness by taking up meditations on
a daily basis, this will decrease the stress levels
that may otherwise hinder proper recognition of
nutritional intake. This might discourage
emotional eating and encourage healthier
options.

14. Calendar or Planner:

You should use a calendar or an organizer for
tracking and organizing your meals, workouts
and any other healthy activity. Such will help you
remain organized and consistent.

15. Sleep and Stress Monitoring:

Take note of the patterns during which you sleep,
as well as how stressed you have been so that you
will be able to determine its influence on your
eating habits and the overall health. They can
therefore be monitored by using apps and
wearables.

It is also important to remember that "it's not
just about numbers." Any issue related to your
emotions, energy levels or overall well-being.
Some quantitative trackers such as self-weighing
may be used while others, mostly qualitative such

as monitoring dietary food intake through food and drink diaries.

**Tips for Maintaining a Commitment to Healthy Eating: **

To stay on the right diet requires hard work sometimes but the above tips will help a person remain focused on his or her health. Here are some tips to help you stay on track:

1. Set clear and realistic goals:

Set reasonable and achievable goals that should help you lose weight. Thus with precisely specified purposes, it gives you an indication of the kind of thing that you want to attain in life.

2. Educate Yourself:

Find out how much nutrition is in your diet. This is a motivation that many people experience in their quest to know how certain food types aid in a person's wellbeing.

3. Meal Planning:

You should cook your meals and snacks a day before. It reduces the possibility of indulging in additional bad choices when one is feeling hungry.

4. Balance and Variety:

Take as many different foods as possible and make sure your diet always consists of protein, carbohydrates, good fats, and fruits and vegetables at any given time.

5. Small, Sustainable Changes:

Do not change your diet dramatically but in steps. On the contrary, it is more likely that smaller, sustainable modifications will fit into life-long habits.

6. Mindful Eating:

Mindful eating means that one should only focus on the taste, feel, and pleasure involved in every morsel.subsection: A number of factors have been used to explain these phenomena. It also aids you in savoring the food and eating mindfully.

7. Stay Hydrated:

At times, people are confused and think that they are hungry instead of thirsty. Drinking enough water during the day will keep you hydrated and avoid the need to snack unnecessarily.

8. Portion Control:

Be mindful of portion sizes. Eating from smaller plates and making correct portion measurements will prevent overeating. #

**9. Keep Healthy Snacks On Hand: **

Have healthy snacks readily available. Always ensure your kitchen is stocked with fruits, vegetables, nuts, and yogurt so that you can reduce the urge of having unhealthy foods.

10. Reward System:

Set up a reward structure for healthier eating. Instead of food rewards, take yourself out for a massage at the spa, buy a new book to read, or even buy yourselves some funky new outfits that will boost your motivation to work out.

11. Accountability:

Divulge your objectives to a close friend or relative for assistance and also to keep you on track.

12. Food Preparation:

Learn how to prepare your meals from scratch and be adventurous about trying out different recipes. Making meals is enjoyable and provides a way of choosing what goes into it as well as controlling the quantities used.

13. Avoid extreme diets:

Stay away from very strict diets which will be difficult to observe for some time. It is a more sustainable approach.

14. Overcome Setbacks:

Do not fail to realize that failure is a step on the path to success. Be gentle with yourself when you occasionally deviate from your plan. Try again, start over and move forward.

15. Seek Inspiration:

Search for a healthy eating and wellness success story on the internet or documentary.

16. Keep a Journal:

Ensure you include these details in your food and mood diary. You will be able to identify the eating pattern as well as emotional attachment that relate to eating disorder problems.

17. Celebrate Small Wins:

Celebrate your successes, no matter how small they are. Enjoy something that you have done, use it as motivation.

18. Positive Self-Talk:

Replace negative self -talk with positive affirmations. Do not lose faith; getting good at something is possible like eating healthy.

19. Exercise Regularly:

Secondly, you can combine them with physical exercises that further boost your motivation.

20. Support System:

Alternatively, you should be part of a support group or an organization of similar people. It has also been found that sharing the experiences and outcome can be motivating and make people feel part of something together.

A pledge to eat healthy always takes time to complete. Some self- care while being observant on routines that have positive implications and you can adhere to it for longer durations.

Keeping a healthy diet and maintaining motivation is hard but manageable with suitable methods. Here are some tips to help you stay on track:

1. Set clear and realistic goals:

Ensure that your healthy eating journey is characterized by realistic goals. Setting goals ensures that you know what to strive for.

**2. Educate Yourself:

Discover what health gains are there in your eating. It can give you motivation in understanding how some foods help and others harm your health.

3. Meal Planning:

Advance plan your meals and snacks. By doing so, it ensures that one will not end up making hurried, unhealthy decisions while hungry.

4. Balance and Variety:

Take different foods as they come up and have well-balanced meals high on proteins, some carbs, some good fat and lots of fruits and veg.

5. Small, Sustainable Changes:

Opt for slow and incremental modifications of your diet rather than drastic dietary replacement. Such small, sustainable adjustments stand higher chances of turning into long-term customs.

6. Mindful Eating:

Eat mindfully by focusing on the food's flavor, feel and entire experience. It enables you to enjoy your food with intentions.

7. Stay Hydrated:

At times, thirst can be misinterpreted as hunger. Take regular sips of water and avoid unwanted munching during the day to remain sufficiently hydrated.

8. Portion Control:

Be mindful of portion sizes. Smaller plates and portion control are effective in preventing overeating.

**9. Keep Healthy Snacks On Hand: **

Have healthy snacks readily available. In the meantime, stock your kitchen with lots of tasty fruits, veggies, nuts and yogurt in order to curb those unhealthy food cravings.

10. Reward System:

Implement a way of rewarding you when you meet your health goals. Indulge in such non-edible gifts as massage, pamphlet, or sports attire.

11. Accountability:

Identify a friend or a family member to share your goals with, and make them responsible for keeping you on track.

12. Food Preparation:

Start cooking and try out new recipes. Planning your own meal is good for you as it gives you a chance of controlling what you consume in large quantities.

13. Avoid extreme diets:

These include avoiding very rigid and unsustainable diets. The way forward should be a balanced strategy.

14. Overcome Setbacks:

Know that these are normal processes in your course and so on. If not often, do not beat yourself up for once in a while straying from your plan. And get back as you go along.

15. Seek Inspiration:

It can involve reading success stories about healthy eating, watching relevant movies, blogs or documentaries.

16. Keep a Journal:

Keep a food and mood diary in order to monitor your progress, difficulties, and achievements.

This will enable you to point out some patterns associated with emotions and food consumption.

17. Celebrate Small Wins:

Do not fail to celebrate any size of success you achieve. Give yourself credit for that effort, and remember that it will motivate you to continue pushing.

18. Positive Self-Talk:

Change the negative self-talk into positive affirmations. Trust yourself, you can eat right.

19. Exercise Regularly:

Additionally, physical activity may serve as an additional incentive and a complimenting effort in maintaining a diet.

20. Support System:

Attend a support group, or find a community. A person may get motivated by such sharing or he/she might feel as a member in progress or experiences.

Keep in mind that keeping to your diet promises is a travel, and not just an end point. Have some patience and focus on cultivating habitual practices which foster overall health in the long run.

Conclusion

If we adopt a balanced diet, self-serve, and mental eating, our bodies will be well fed for good performance. Portion control makes it possible for us to eat what our bodies require without overeating thus preventing related morbidities. Starting with a balanced plate containing colorful fruits and vegetables, lean proteins, complex carbs, and good fats becomes key for maintaining a vibrant life.